VICTORIAN LIFE

A VICTORIAN
HOSPITAL

KATRINA SILIPRANDI

Wayland

VICTORIAN LIFE

A VICTORIAN CHRISTMAS

A VICTORIAN FACTORY

A VICTORIAN HOLIDAY

A VICTORIAN HOSPITAL

A VICTORIAN KITCHEN

A VICTORIAN SCHOOL

A VICTORIAN STREET

A VICTORIAN SUNDAY

A VICTORIAN WORKHOUSE

VICTORIAN CLOTHES

VICTORIAN TOYS AND GAMES

VICTORIAN TRANSPORT

HOW WE LEARN ABOUT THE VICTORIANS

Queen Victoria reigned from 1837 to 1901, a time when Britain went through enormous social and industrial changes. We can learn about the Victorians in various ways. We can still see many of their buildings standing today and we can look at their documents, maps and artefacts – many of which can be found in museums. Photography, invented during Victoria's reign, gives us a good picture of life in Victorian Britain. In this book you will see what Victorian life was like through some of this historical evidence.

Series design: Pardoe Blacker Ltd
Editors: Sarah Doughty and Katie Orchard
Production controller: Carol Stevens

First published in 1994 by Wayland (Publishers) Ltd,
61 Western Road, Hove, East Sussex BN3 1JD, England

© Copyright 1994 Wayland (Publishers) Ltd

British Library Cataloguing in Publication Data
Siliprandi, Katrina
  Victorian Hospital. – (Victorian Life Series)
  I. Title II. Series
  362.10941

ISBN 0 7502 1263 2

Printed and bound in Great Britain by B.P.C.
Paulton Books

Cover picture: A picture of a ward in St. Bartholomew's hospital in London.

Picture acknowledgements:
The Beamish Museum 24; The Bridgeman Art Library 17 (top); Mary Evans 5 (bottom), 8, 15, 16, 17 (bottom), 21(top), 22, 23 (top and bottom), 26 (top); Guildhall Library 26 (bottom); The Hulton Deutsch Collection 18 and 19 (top), 25 (bottom); Image Select 6 (top); Leeds City Council 4; Natural History Picture Agency 9 (bottom); Ann Ronan Picture Library 6 (bottom), 7; The Science Museum 9 (top), 10 (top and bottom), 11, 12, 13 (top), 14 (top and bottom), 18 (bottom), 19 (bottom), 20; Strathclyde Regional Council 27; The Wellcome Institute Library *cover,* 5 (top), 13 (bottom), 21 (bottom), 25 (top) © Copyright King's College Hospital.

With special thanks to the Science Museum for the commissioned pictures that appear in the book.

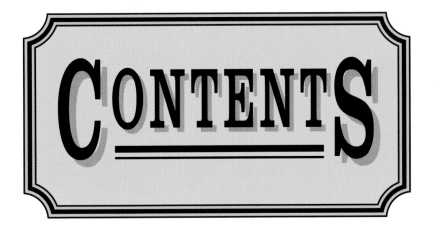

CONTENTS

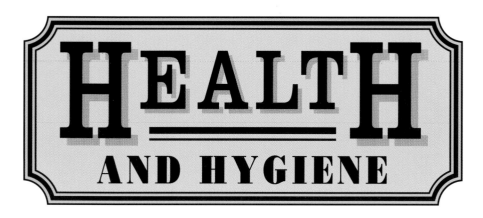

HEALTH AND HYGIENE

In the hundred years before Queen Victoria's reign began in 1837, industry in Britain had begun to develop. This changed the lives of many people. New factories had been built and towns had become much bigger as people moved from the countryside and came to look for jobs in the new factory towns.

A view of Leeds in 1846.

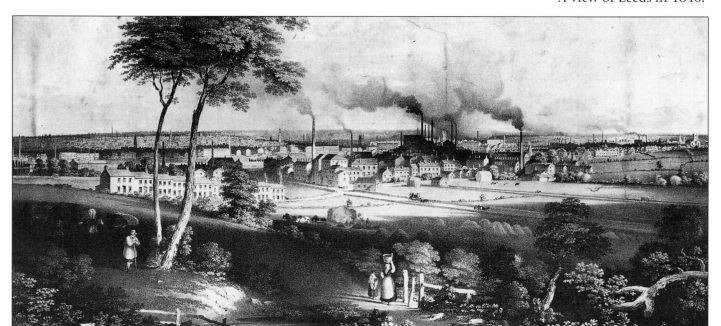

UNHEALTHY CONDITIONS

Most people in towns like Leeds lived in poor conditions in early Victorian Britain. Houses were built very close together so they did not have much light or ventilation. Rubbish was thrown into the streets or the rivers. People did not have piped water or taps in their homes. Water was collected from streams or rivers into which sewers drained. Some people had to share a tap or pump in the street.

WASTE DISPOSAL

The notice on the right warned people in Clerkenwell, London, that a disease called cholera was coming. Diseases spread quickly in the unhealthy conditions in the towns. Most people did not have toilets that flushed. They used outdoor privies above cesspits. The foul-smelling cesspits were emptied after dark by night men. The night men tipped what they had collected into huge cesspits or emptied them on to dung heaps. These were often close to houses.

In Greenock, Scotland, a local doctor reported:

'In one part of Market Street is a dunghill, yet it is too large to be called a dunghill...it contains 100 cubic yards [76 cubic metres] of impure filth!'

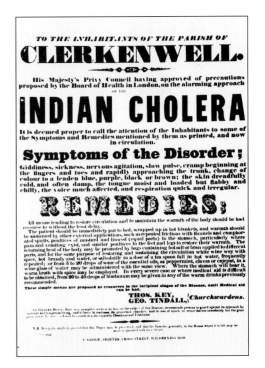

A notice to warn people of the spread of cholera.

THE SPREAD OF CHOLERA

Unhygienic living conditions.

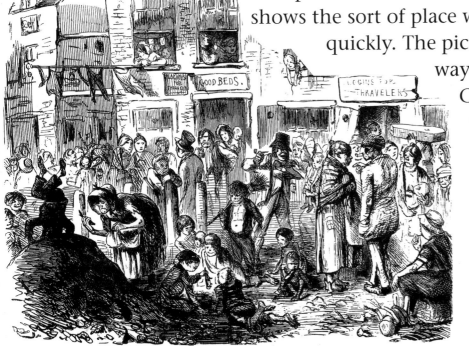

This picture is called *A Court for King Cholera*. It shows the sort of place where diseases spread very quickly. The picture illustrates different ways of spreading disease. Children are playing among the mice and rats. A woman is rooting through the dirty rubbish. The rubbish and waste is piled up in the street. We know today that all of these things would have been quite dangerous to people's health.

FATAL DISEASES

This person is dying from cholera. Someone with cholera would have suffered terribly. He or she went blue in the face and had attacks of cramp, sickness and diarrhoea. Cholera killed half the people who caught it. There were other diseases that killed people in Victorian times, such as typhus, tuberculosis, measles and whooping cough. People thought that diseases spread in two ways. One idea was that an illness was caught by touching someone who already had it. The other idea was that diseases were spread by miasma. This was the bad smells from filth in the streets, privies and drains. These diseases sometimes spread to rich people, so they wanted to find out how to stop them.

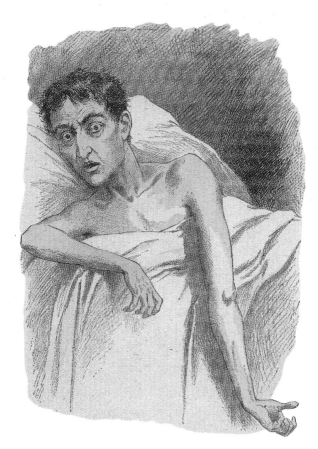

A cholera victim.

CHILD DEATH

These parents are looking at the gravestone which marks where their child is buried. One out of every five babies born in 1880 died before he or she was one year old. Poor people who lived in the country lived twice as long as poor people who lived in the towns. This was because the air was clearer, there were fewer people to spread diseases and people's homes were not so close together.

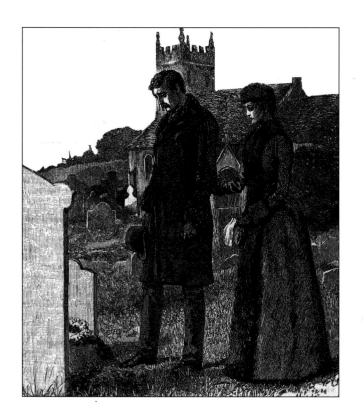

Parents at a gravestone, 1888.

AMPUTATION

Some people's illnesses became worse because of the medical treatment they received. In some serious medical cases, parts of the body became infected and the only course of action was to amputate. The patient in this picture is about to have his arm cut off at the shoulder. The surgeon is the man wearing an apron and holding a knife, while his assistant holds the patient still. The surgeon was probably wearing his oldest, dirtiest clothes because he did not understand about germs. We know now that many illnesses are caused by germs.

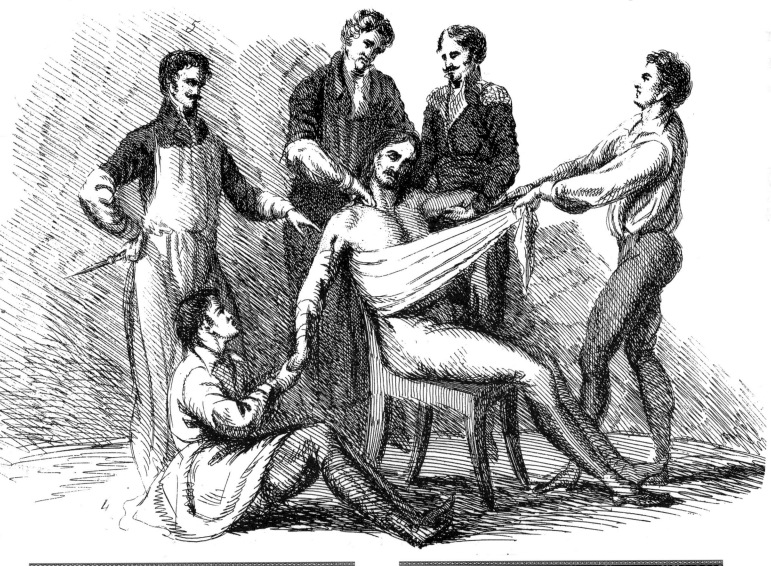

A patient about to have his arm amputated.

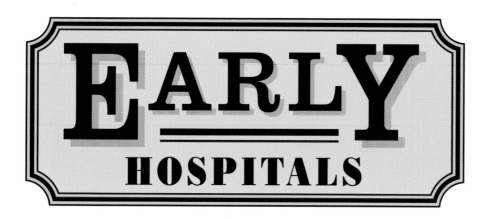

EARLY HOSPITALS

At the start of Queen Victoria's reign, hospitals were for poor people. Rich people were treated by doctors at home. People who went into hospital often did not come out again alive. They caught diseases from other patients or they died from the treatment they were given.

HOSPITAL CONDITIONS

This was a hospital ward in 1808. People with different illnesses were all in the same room. In early Victorian Britain there were two kinds of hospitals. Voluntary hospitals were one type, which were run using money given by rich people. The other type of hospital was a workhouse, which also had wards called infirmaries for sick people. Nurses in voluntary hospitals worked long hours. They slept in rooms that were described as 'wooden cages on the landing'.

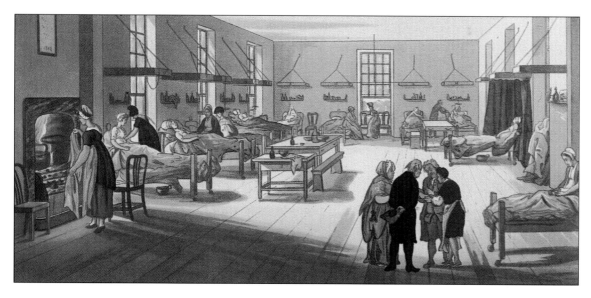

Middlesex Hospital in 1808.

Only poor women became nurses. They had no medical knowledge. Hospitals were dirty and smelled bad. The patients and staff used buckets on the wards for toilets. Here is a description of a hospital: 'Filth was universal. The patients wore the same shirt for seven weeks; bedding was only changed and washed once a month; food was at starvation level.'

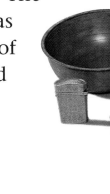

A leech jar, bowls and blades.

'BAD BLOOD'

Doctors thought many illnesses were caused by 'bad' or poisoned blood. To get rid of the poisons the patient was cut with a knife or blade like the ones at the front of the picture. The blood was collected in a bowl. Blood was measured using the lines on the inside of the bowl. These numbered lines showed how much blood had been collected. Leeches were sometimes used to collect blood. They were kept in a leech jar.

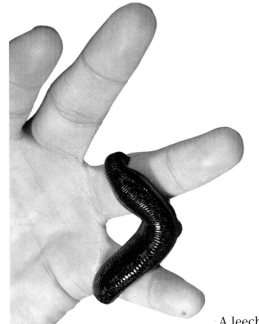

A leech on a patient's hand.

LEECHES

Putting leeches on to a patient's skin was a popular way of getting the blood out of the patients. This picture shows how the leeches sucked the blood. Infectious diseases, growths and even broken bones were treated in this way, as medical knowledge at the time was very limited.

A SURGEON'S TOOLS

This picture shows the tools a Victorian surgeon would have used for operations. They include saws and knives. In early Victorian times, operations were very dangerous. This was because there were no drugs to put the patients to sleep. Also, doctors did not understand that wounds should be kept clean and equipment should be sterilized. The most usual operation was to cut off a part of the body, like an arm or a leg. This could be done very quickly using a saw.

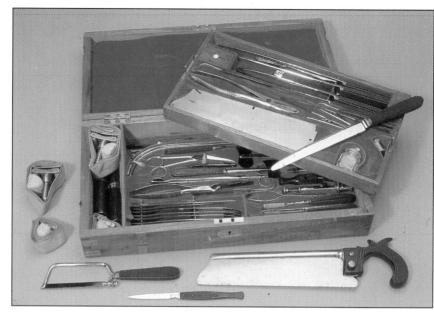

Some of the tools a surgeon would have used.

OPERATIONS

Operations were done on a wooden table covered with a cloth. The surgeon probably wore an old coat covered with blood and pus. His instruments were not sterilized. The patient was given a piece of leather to bite on when the pain became too great. Many patients probably screamed. There was sawdust on the floor to collect dripping blood. After the operation, a dressing like the one in the picture might have been put on the wound. A man who had had his foot cut off wrote: 'Of the agony it occasioned I will say nothing. Suffering so great as I underwent cannot be expressed in words...'

A dressing.

Even when patients survived these operations, many died soon afterwards from blood poisoning or shock. Rich people did not go into hospital. If they had to have an operation, it was done by a doctor on the kitchen table at home.

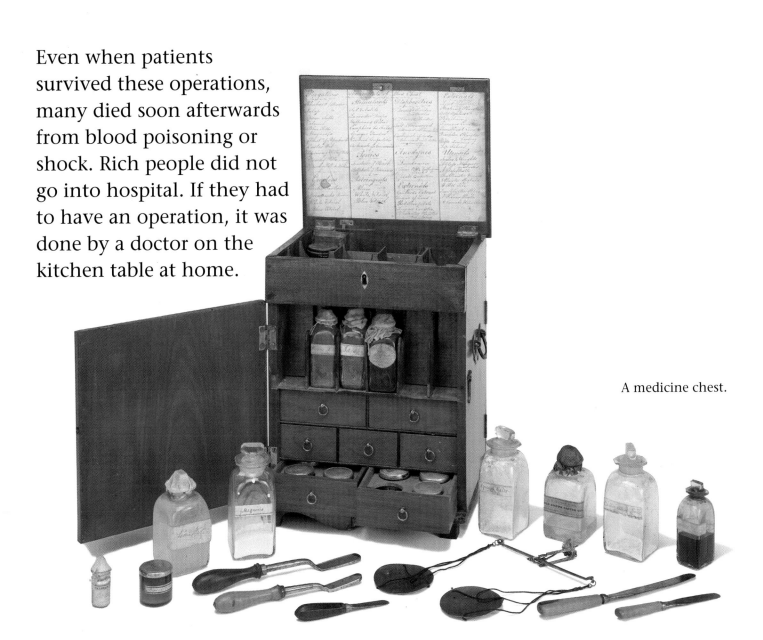

A medicine chest.

EARLY MEDICINES

Medicines like the ones in the picture were usually made from plants or minerals. Some drugs were actually quite harmful. A drug called opium, made from poppies, was often used to stop pain. Once people were given opium they became addicted to it and found it hard to live without. For some illnesses, a substance called canthandine was used. This comes from crushed beetles. It was put on to the skin and cloth was wrapped around it. It made the skin blister. Doctors thought that blood would rush to the sore blister, away from the injured area, and the patient would recover.

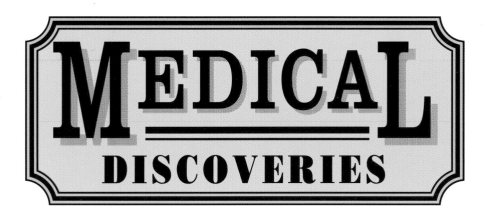

MEDICAL DISCOVERIES

A drug that is used to put someone to sleep is called an anaesthetic. Ether was first used as an anaesthetic in 1846. Ether is a liquid that produces a gas which is a good painkiller. But it made patients cough and vomit and it could be dangerous. Dr Simpson (1811–1870) at Edinburgh University experimented with other gases. In 1847 he discovered that chloroform was a good anaesthetic.

ANAESTHETICS

A mask like the one in the picture, soaked in chloroform, was put over the patient's face. The patient breathed in the chloroform and went to sleep. Some people thought it was wrong to use anaesthetics. They believed it was natural to feel pain. Queen Victoria used chloroform to kill the pain of childbirth when her son was born in 1853. When her ninth baby was due in 1857, she said: 'We are having this baby and we are having chloroform'. After that, the use of anaesthetics was widely accepted.

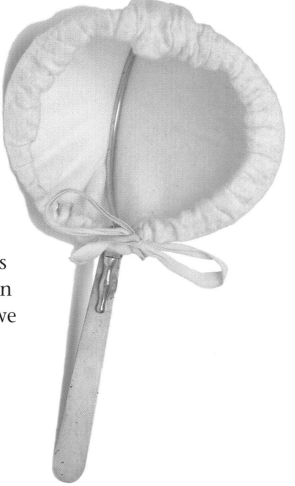

A chloroform mask.

DRUGS FOR OPERATIONS

Hypodermic syringes, like the one in the picture, were invented in 1853. They could be used to inject drugs like morphine, another anaesthetic. From about 1884, cocaine was also used to stop pain. Anaesthetics were very important because they meant surgeons could work more carefully and slowly. They could carry out more difficult operations. However, many patients still died from infections caused by germs. In 1869, two out of every five patients died after their operation.

A hypodermic syringe and case.

DISINFECTANTS

In 1864 a French chemist called Louis Pasteur (1822–1895) proved that infections were caused by germs. A surgeon in Glasgow called Joseph Lister (1827–1912) used this knowledge to invent a spray. It sent a fine mist of the disinfectant carbolic acid into the air while he was operating. This spray was used to kill germs that might infect the patient during the operation.

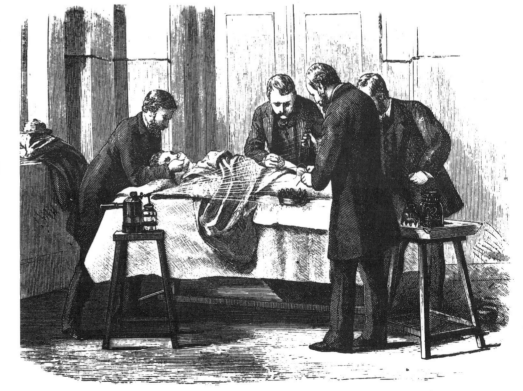

Lister's handspray being used in an operation in 1882.

STERILIZING EQUIPMENT

Lister also soaked his hands and instruments in carbolic acid. He covered wounds in disinfected bandages. Many people did not think that Lister's ideas were right. They felt that it was all a waste of time and did not even believe that germs existed, because they could not see them.

However, Lister's ideas were accepted during the 1880s. In time it was realized that the best way to stop infections was to prevent germs from getting near the patient. Robert Koch (1843–1910), a German bacteriologist, discovered that hot steam killed more germs than disinfectant. New medical instruments were all made out of metal so they could be boiled. Surgeons wore rubber gloves from about 1890 and gauze face-masks were first worn in 1899.

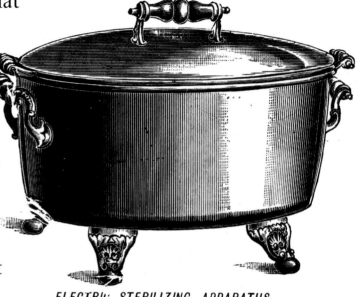

ELECTRIC STERILIZING APPARATUS.

An advertisement for sterilizing equipment.

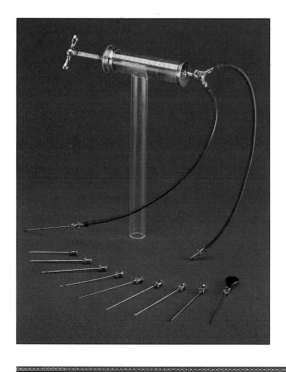

An aspirator.

TREATMENT FOR TUBERCULOSIS

In the nineteenth century, tuberculosis was a common disease that killed most people who caught it. A new discovery was made which could help to cure it. It was called an aspirator and was used to drain liquid from a person's lungs. This helped people with tuberculosis to breathe more easily. The germ that caused tuberculosis was discovered by Koch in 1882.

IMPROVED HYGIENE

During Queen Victoria's reign, laws were passed to try and make towns cleaner and healthier. By 1900 Britain had many new, clean water supplies. Cholera no longer existed in Britain. Some factory owners built good homes for their workers. Many houses had toilets that flushed, but several families often shared one toilet. The pumping station in this picture was built in 1868. It was part of a new sewerage system for London.

Abbey Mills Pumping Station in 1868.

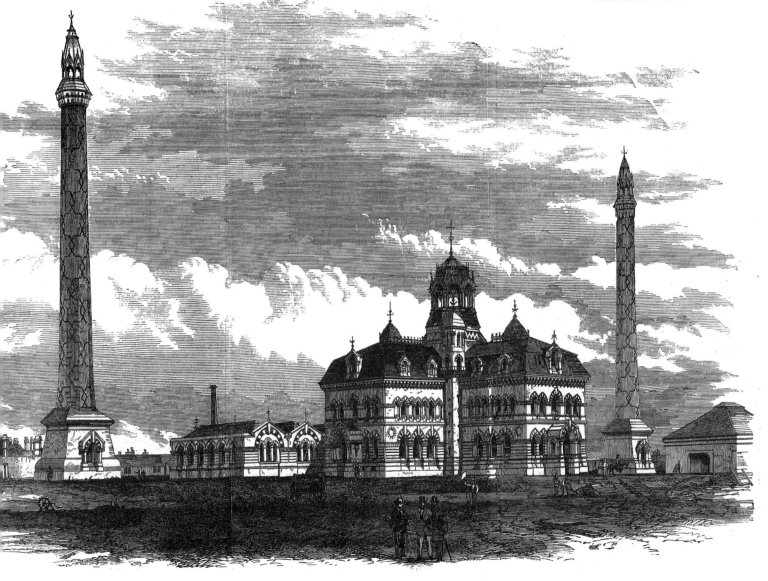

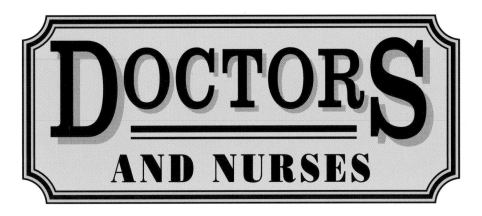

DOCTORS AND NURSES

In early Victorian times it was realized that doctors needed proper training. In 1858 a law was passed which meant that only qualified people could work as doctors. Schools were set up to give this new training. There were also improvements in training nurses in the nineteenth century.

UNQUALIFIED SURGEONS

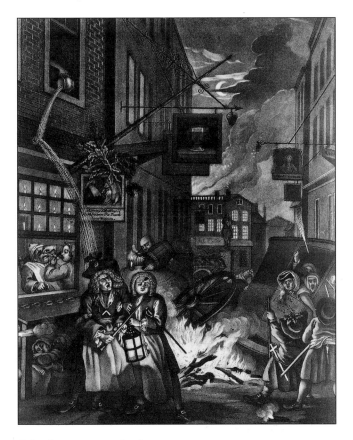

A barber-surgeon's shop.

Before 1800, small operations were carried out by barber-surgeons. You can see one at work in the picture on the left, from 1738. Training for surgeons was set up in the eighteenth century, but many doctors were still unqualified when Victoria came to the throne. A writer called Edward Harrison found that in three small towns in Britain: 'sixty-nine persons practise medicine for money in this area of whom not one in nine has been educated for the profession!'

A law called the Medical Act was passed in 1858. It was important because it said what education and qualifications a doctor must have.

FLORENCE NIGHTINGALE

Florence Nightingale (1820–1910) came from a rich family. Her family was shocked when she decided to train as a nurse in Germany. In 1854 British soldiers were fighting the Crimean War. The conditions in the hospital for wounded soldiers in Scutari, near the Black Sea, were dreadful. Nightingale wanted to help. She went to Scutari with thirty-eight nurses. They worked very hard and improved things. You can see how clean the hospital was after Florence Nightingale arrived.

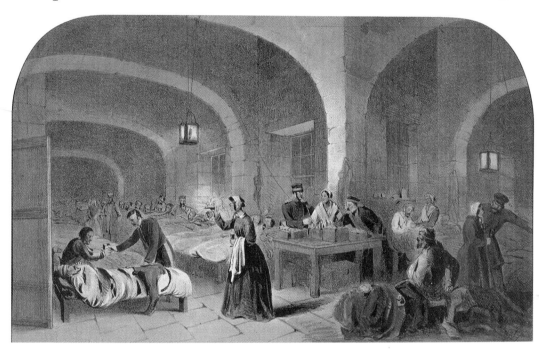

Scutari after Florence Nightingale decided to help.

MARY SEACOLE

Mary Seacole travelled from Jamaica to help the soldiers in the Crimea. She had heard of the terrible conditions that the soldiers were living in and decided to help the wounded men out there. She opened a rest home for soldiers, with good food and medicines. Mary Seacole was very brave. She even went out on to the battlefield to help the wounded.

Mary Seacole (1803–81).

TRAINING NURSES

When Nightingale came back from the Crimea, she set up a training school for nurses at St. Thomas's Hospital. The training lasted a year. It was strict. Nurses lived at the hospital and were only allowed to go outside its walls in pairs. Part of their training at the hospital was to learn some Latin so that they could read the labels on medicine bottles. Gradually, other hospitals also set up training schools for nurses. By the 1890s nursing was seen as a suitable job for women. It was no longer only poor people who became nurses. In 1901 there were 68,000 trained nurses in Britain. In 1850 there had been none.

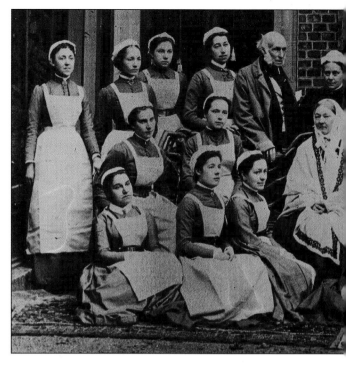

Florence Nightingale and a group of nurses.

TRAINING DOCTORS

A model of an operating theatre in 1895.

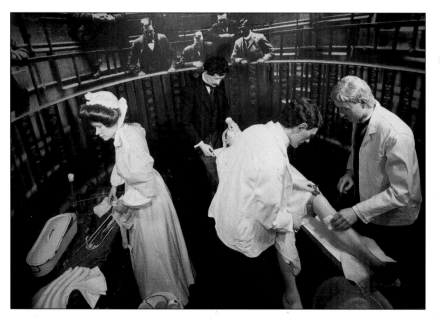

This is how an operating theatre looked in 1895. In the hospitals with training schools, trainee doctors could watch operations and learn from experienced doctors. Women were allowed to train as doctors, from 1876. In late Victorian times, surgeons could carry out many operations. They could operate on the stomach, bladder and kidneys. The first successful removal of an appendix was done in 1880.

THE CHEMIST'S SHOP

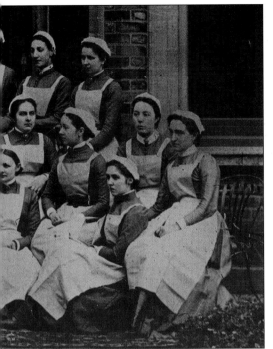

Here you can see a chemist's shop as it might have looked in 1901. Knowledge about medicines increased in Victorian times. In late Victorian times you could buy many different medicines, like Beechams pills, Doctor Williams' Pink Pills for Pale People, and Boots No-Name Ointment. Aspirin was first sold in shops in 1899.

A reconstruction of a chemist's shop in 1901.

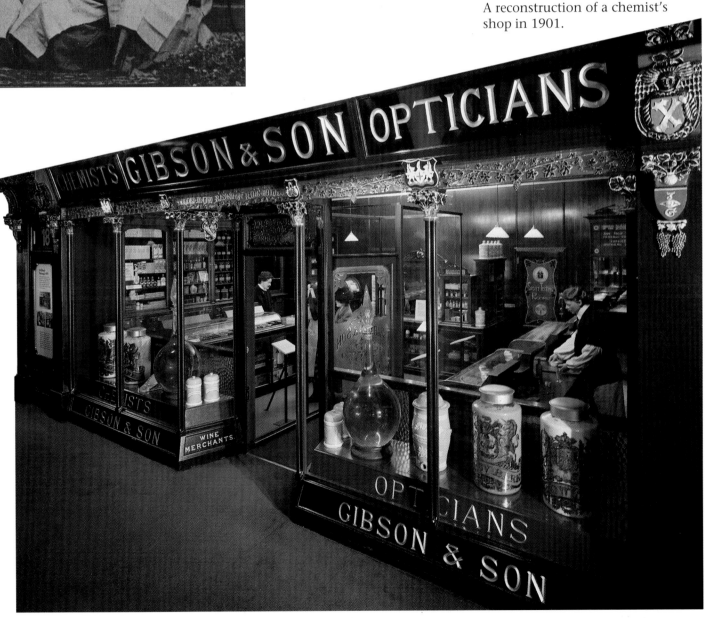

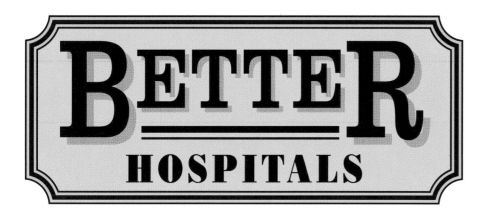

BETTER HOSPITALS

During Queen Victoria's reign, hospitals changed and improved. Many new hospitals were built. Some hospitals had schools where doctors and nurses trained. They were often the places where discoveries were made and new treatments were tried. Some hospitals began to specialize in certain areas of medicine.

BETTER EQUIPMENT

In late Victorian times, several important inventions were developed and doctors had better equipment. The ophthalmoscope was invented in 1851. This could be used to see the back of a patient's eye. The respirator in the picture gave patients oxygen if they had breathing difficulties. Four patients could use it at once. In 1880 an instrument for measuring blood pressure was invented.

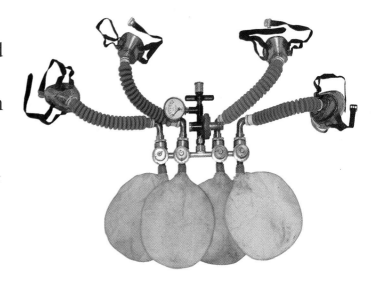

An oxygen respirator.

DOCTOR'S ROUNDS

In this picture, doctors are visiting the patients in hospital. Some of the men are probably still learning to be doctors. Some medical conditions were not treated in hospitals. For instance, at the end of Queen Victoria's reign almost all babies were born at home. Poor women usually had midwives to help them to have their baby. Midwives often had no medical training. They knew what to do from experience. Richer women usually had a doctor to help them. The doctor often knew very little about childbirth. In Victorian times, rich women were more likely to die in childbirth than poor women.

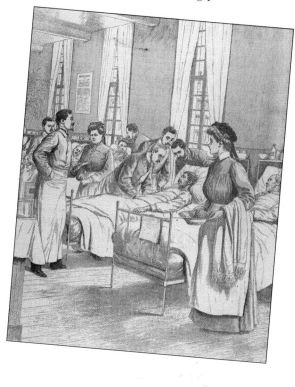

Doctors visiting patients.

SPECIALIST HOSPITALS

In this hospital, boys are in the same ward as men. In 1850 there were few hospitals especially for children, despite the high death rate among young children and babies. In London nearly half of the people who died were under ten years old. In 1852, Dr West opened the London Hospital for Sick Children in Great Ormond Street. Children's hospitals were later set up in other towns in Britain.

Other specialist hospitals started in Victorian times. In London the Ear, Nose and Throat Hospital opened in 1838 and the London Skin Hospital opened in 1887. They were important because they allowed doctors to find out more about one kind of illness.

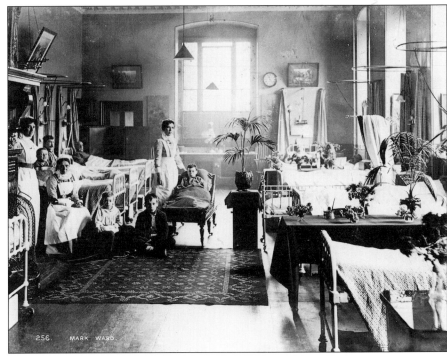

A ward in St. Bartholomew's Hospital in London.

FAIRHAM COMMUNITY COLLEGE

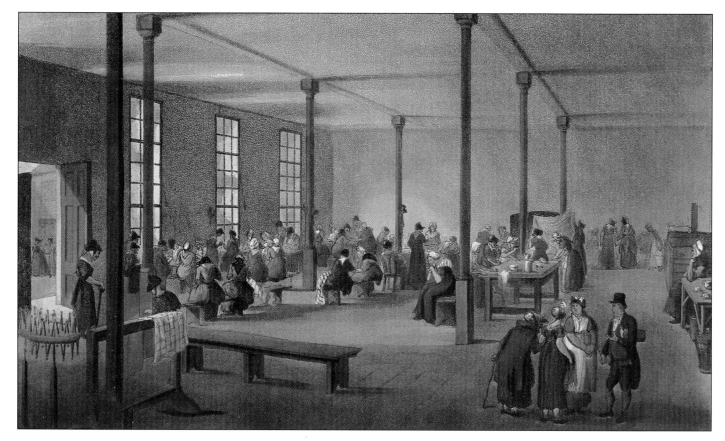

An early nineteenth-century workhouse.

WORKHOUSES

This is a workhouse in the early nineteenth century. The conditions in workhouse infirmaries were even worse than in other hospitals. There was no proper medical or nursing care. A workhouse ward was usually made up of helpless, bedridden patients with poor, untrained nurses to help them.

In Liverpool in 1865, trained nurses were used in the new workhouse infirmary for the first time. They improved conditions for the patients so much that in Liverpool it became the rule to use trained nurses. Later, other workhouse hospitals did the same.

In country areas some doctors set up small hospitals for patients who could afford to pay. They were called cottage hospitals. They only had a few beds. By 1900 there were over 300 cottage hospitals in Britain.

MENTAL ILLNESS

In Victorian times people who were mentally ill were kept in special hospitals called asylums. Some patients were chained up to keep them under control. Gradually, however, people came to understand that these patients did not have to be chained up to control them and that they were not dangerous. There were laws passed to improve conditions in asylums.

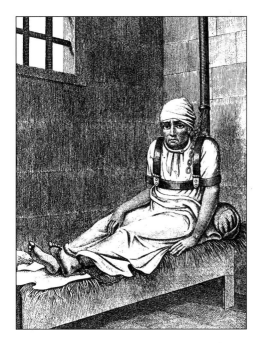

A patient in an asylum.

DOCTOR'S FEES

These people are waiting to see a doctor. In 1881 a visit to the doctor cost between $12\frac{1}{2}$p and $37\frac{1}{2}$p in today's money. At the time a baker was paid about £1.00 a week and a hairdresser was paid about 50p a week. So a doctor's visit could take up a large part of the average weekly wage. For many families a visit from the doctor was a luxury which they could not afford.

A doctor's waiting room.

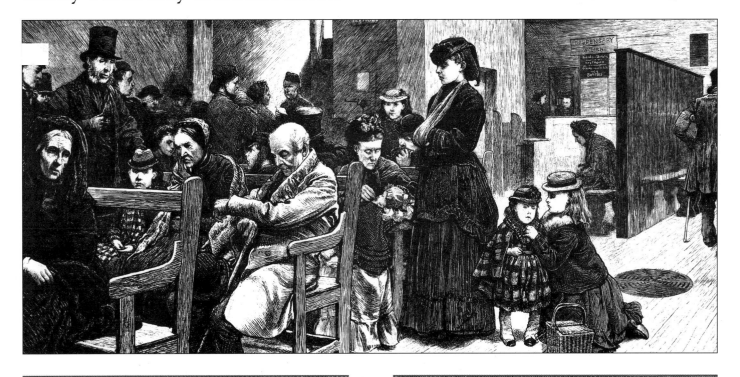

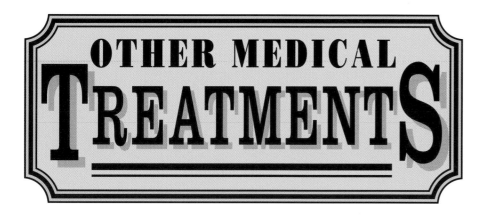

OTHER MEDICAL TREATMENTS

By the end of Queen Victoria's reign, knowledge about surgery, medicine and health had changed a great deal. All areas of medical treatment had improved, and hospitals could provide better help and health care. Even dentists were able to use the new medical discoveries in their work. These changes, however, did not always happen quickly.

DENTISTS

This is how a dentist's surgery might have looked in the 1890s. You can see the bottles of gas used as an anaesthetic. By this time dentists had to be trained. Things were very different in early Victorian times. Many dentists were unqualified tooth-pullers. They travelled from town to town and pulled out teeth for anyone who could pay. Before 1845, false teeth were made from gold or real teeth from dead people. Later, porcelain teeth were made. Only rich people could afford them. When vulcanite was discovered in about 1870, false teeth became cheaper.

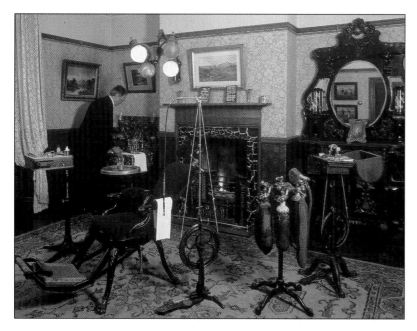

A dentist's surgery.

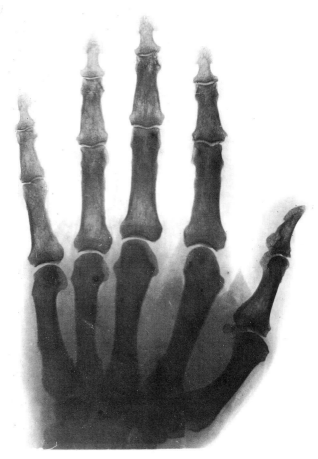

X-RAYS

In 1895 a German scientist called Wilhelm Röntgen (1845–1923) found out about X-rays. He used X-rays to take photographs of the inside of the body. This picture shows the first X-ray that was ever taken. It is Röntgen's wife's hand. At first, X-rays were used to look at broken bones. Today they can also be used to help doctors find out about many different illnesses.

An X-ray of a hand.

RADIUM

Near the end of Victorian times, another important discovery was made. Two French scientists, Marie and Pierre Curie (1867–1937 and 1859–1906) discovered a metal called radium in 1898. It was used to treat cancer and is still used today. Radium is quite dangerous in large amounts. Marie Curie died from radium burns, but her discovery has helped many other people to live longer.

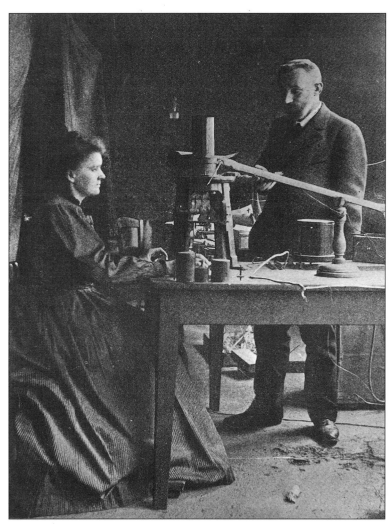

Marie and Pierre Curie.

CORSETS

Women wore corsets like these in Victorian Britain. It was thought that corsets would help strengthen their spines and keep their organs strong and healthy. They were also meant to give women a graceful figure. This advertisement says that wearing a corset like this is good for you. In fact, many women damaged themselves by fastening the corset too tightly.

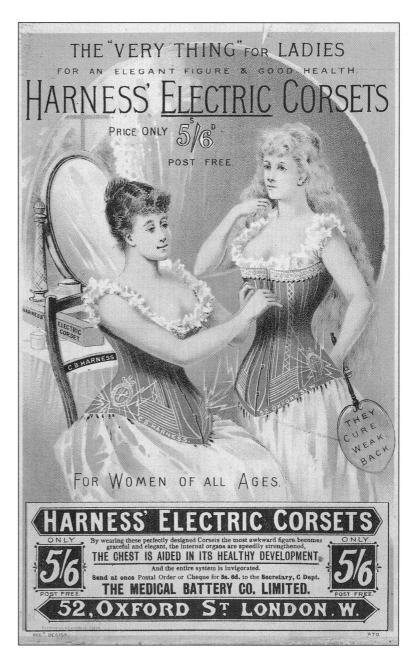

A corset advertisement.

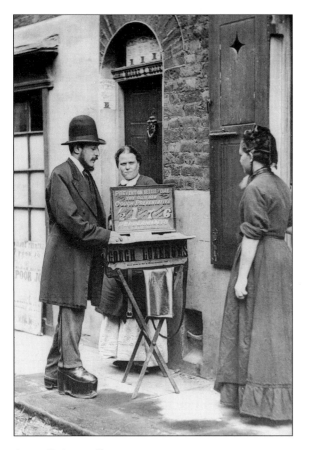

A medicine seller.

OTHER REMEDIES

Most people in Victorian Britain could not afford to see the doctor. Some people bought medicines from street sellers or chemist shops. Some of the medicines were no good. Holloway's pills claimed to cure many illnesses. In fact they were just 'butter, lard, turps, wax and nothing else'!

The most common treatments were home-made medicines. Onions, vinegar and brown sugar were used to make cough medicine. Grated acorns were used for diarrhoea. Brown paper soaked in vinegar was used for headaches. Breathing in the air near a gasworks was wrongly thought to be a cure for whooping cough.

HOW THINGS CHANGED

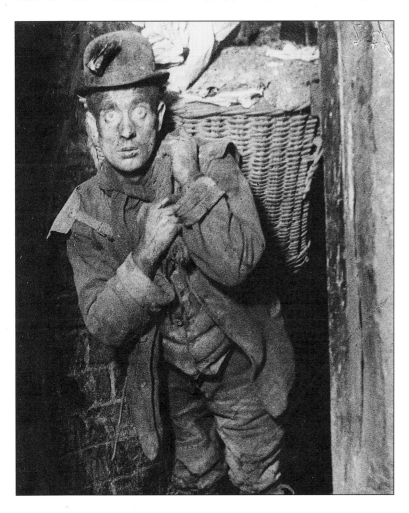

A Glasgow street-cleaner.

In this book you have found out how much things changed in Victorian Britain. Street-cleaners like this one and clean water supplies made towns healthier. However, many people still lived in overcrowded homes. Hospitals improved and were much safer, and doctors knew more about diseases. Yet there were many illnesses that they could not cure. People still had to pay to go to hospital or to see a doctor, and many could not afford to pay. In general, people were still very unhealthy. For instance, in 1899 more soldiers were needed to fight the Boer War. In one town only one out of every ten men was found to be well enough. Out of every 1,000 babies born at the end of Queen Victoria's reign, 163 died before they were one year old. Clearly, there was still a long way to go.

TIME LINE

1830s

1837 Queen Victoria's reign started.

1838 Metropolitan Ear, Nose and Throat Hospital opened.

1839 Sanitary Commission founded.

1840s

1840 Kensington Children's Hospital opened.

1847 Dr Simpson first used chloroform as an anaesthetic.

1848 Cholera and Public Health Act.

1848–9 Cholera epidemic in Britain.

1850s

1850 London Smallpox Hospital opened.

1852 Great Ormond Street Hospital for Sick Children opened.

1853 Queen Victoria accepted chloroform during childbirth.

Hypodermic syringes invented.

1854–7 Crimean War.

1858 Royal Dental Hospital opened.

Medical Act.

1859 Cranleigh Hospital opened one of the first cottage hospitals.

1860s

1860 Nightingale set up a training school for nurses at St. Thomas's Hospital.

1864 Lister used carbolic spray.

1864 Louis Pasteur proved that infections are caused by germs.

1866 Sanitary Act. Every town had to appoint a sanitary inspector. Inspectors could stop landlords overcrowding their premises and force them to remove health hazards.

| 1066 | | 1485 | 1603 | 1714 | 1837 | 1901 |

MIDDLE AGES

NORMANS

TUDORS

STUARTS

GEORGIANS

VICTORIANS

20TH CENTURY

1870s

1874 London School of Medicine founded.

1875 Second Public Health Act. There had to be a Public Health Committee in every area. It had to provide water, sewage and rubbish clearance and inspect food and markets.

1876 General Medical Council admitted women to the Medical Register so they could become doctors.

1876 Dentists Act. Dentists had to be registered and have proper training, like doctors.

1880s

1880 Instrument for measuring blood pressure invented.

First successful removal of an appendix.

1880–2 Carl Joseph Eberth found the germ that caused typhus.

1882 Robert Koch found the germ that caused tuberculosis.

c.1884 Cocaine used as an anaesthetic.

1887 London Skin Hospital opened.

1890s

c.1890 Surgical gloves worn for the first time.

1895 Wilhelm Röntgen discovered X-rays.

1896 First open-heart surgery performed.

1898 Marie Curie discovered radium.

1899 Aspirin first sold in shops.

Gauze face masks first worn for operations.

1899–1902 Boer War.

1900s

1900 Karl Landsteiner demonstrated that not all human blood was the same. He discovered at least three types.

1901 Death of Queen Victoria.

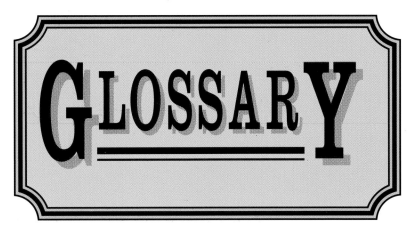

GLOSSARY

Anaesthetic A drug used to put a person, or a part of the body, to sleep so that pain cannot be felt.

Asylum A place where mentally ill people were kept.

Barber-surgeon A man who shaved people, pulled out teeth and let blood.

Carbolic acid A liquid which kills germs. It is used as an antiseptic or disinfectant.

Cesspit A pit for privies and dirty water to drain into.

Chloroform A type of anaesthetic.

Cholera A disease caused by germs in water or food.

Cocaine A drug which was used as an anaesthetic.

Cottage hospital A small hospital, sometimes in a cottage. Cottage hospitals were set up in the countryside by doctors for patients who could pay.

Disease Illness or sickness.

Disinfect To free from germs and sterilize.

Dung Manure.

Ether An early type of anaesthetic.

Gauze A thin, transparent fabric.

Hypodermic A fine, hollow needle used to inject drugs under the skin, into the blood stream.

Infection An illness caused by germs.

Latin The language of ancient Rome. Medical terms are in Latin.

Leech A blood-sucking worm.

Miasma A nasty smell polluting the atmosphere.

Midwife Someone who helps with the birth of a baby.

Morphine A very strong anaesthetic.

Ophthalmoscope An instrument for looking at the back of the eyes.

Porcelain A type of china.

Privy A toilet that does not flush. Usually a hole in the ground.

Pus A yellow liquid found in sores.

Radium A radioactive metal found in minerals. It was discovered by Marie Curie and is still used to treat cancer today.

Sterile Clinically clean and without germs.

Stethoscope An instrument used for hearing the sounds inside the body.

Syringe An instrument for squirting and injecting, used with a hypodermic needle.

Tuberculosis An infectious illness mostly affecting the lungs.

Typhus An infectious disease caused by germs. Symptoms usually include high fever, skin rash and severe headaches.

Ventilation A good, clean air supply.

Vulcanite A kind of rubber.

Whooping cough An infectious disease which results in a severe cough.

Workhouse A place for poor, old or sick people who had nowhere else to go.

BOOKS TO READ

For older readers:

Bartley, P. and Bourdillon, H. *Modern Medicine* (Edward Arnold, 1989)

Historical books:

Baly, M. E. *Nursing, Past and Present* (Batsford, 1981)

Evans, D. *How we used to live, Victorians Early and Late* (A & C Black, 1990)

Hodgson, P. *Nursing* (Batsford, 1986)

Morgan, N. *Life Stories: Florence Nightingale* (Wayland, 1992)

Mountfield, A. *Looking Back at Medicine* (Macdonald Education Ltd, 1988)

Parker, S. *History of Medicine* (Belitha Press, 1991)

Rawcliffe, M. *Finding Out About Victorian Towns* (Batsford, 1982)

Tames, R. *Florence Nightingale* (Franklin Watts, 1989)

Wood, S. *Living in Victorian Times* (John Murray, 1985)

Twentieth-century medicine:

Bryan, J. *Medicine in the Twentieth Century* (Wayland, 1988)

PLACES TO VISIT

Many museums have displays about Victorian medicine. Here are just a few of them.

ENGLAND

London: The Florence Nightingale Museum, 2 Lambeth Palace Road, London SE1 7EW. Tel: 071-620 0374.

Guards Museum, Wellington Barracks, London, SW1E 6HQ. Tel: 071-414 3271.

The Royal London Hospital Archive and Museum, Church of St. Augustine with St. Philip, Newark Street, London SE1 6HQ. Tel: 071-377 700.

The Science Museum, Exhibition Road, London, SW7 2DD, Tel: 071-938 8000.

Yorkshire: The Medical Museum, 131 Beckett Street, Leeds, LS9 7LP. Tel: 0532-444 343.

SCOTLAND

Edinburgh: Museum of the Royal College of Surgeons of Edinburgh, 18 Nicholson Street, Edinburgh, EH8 9DW.

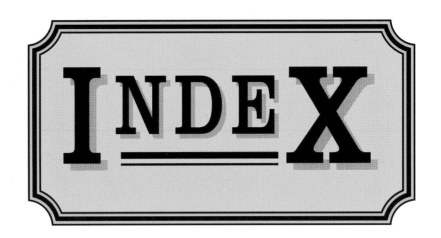

INDEX